The *Wholeness Quest*
Workbook & Journal

Reflections on the 10 signposts of the
Heroine's Journey

Veronica Strachan

True Dialogue
Publishing

Copyright © 2020 Veronica Strachan

All rights reserved.

The author would like to acknowledge the Wurundjeri people who are the Traditional Custodians of the Land on which she lives, and pay her respects to Elders past, present, and emerging of the Kulin Nation, and to all other Indigenous Australians who have been telling their stories for tens of thousands of years.

American readers please note, this workbook and journal uses Australian spelling.

The author of this book does not dispense medical advice or prescribe the use of any technique as a form of treatment for physical, emotional, or medical problems without the advice of a qualified medical or other health professional, either directly or indirectly.

The intent of the author is only to offer information of a general nature to help you in your quest for emotional and spiritual well-being. In the event you use any of the information in this book for yourself, which is your right, the author assumes no responsibility for your actions.

First published 2020 by Veronica Eileen Strachan

True Dialogue Publishing

Cover and women figures designed and drawn by Cassi Strachan of Creative Girl Tuesday

Paperback ISBN-13: 978-0-6485134-6-9

Ebook ISBN-13: 978-0-6485134-8-3

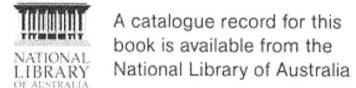

Dedicated to all the wonderful women in my life

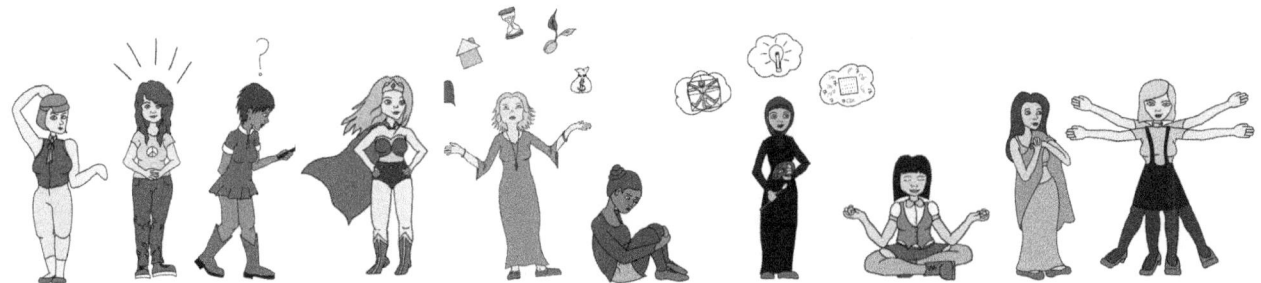

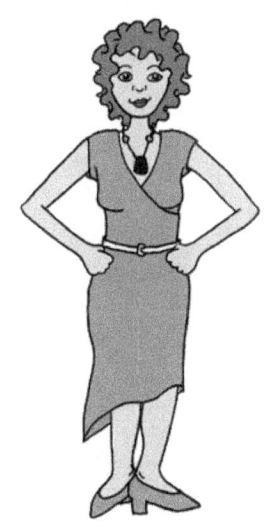

Contents

Behind the 10 signposts of my Heroine's Journey	1
A word on journalling before you begin	6
How to use this workbook & journal	8
1. Conflicted and confused?	10
Starting a gratitude journal	12
30-day gratitude challenge	16
2. Conscious	30
Exploring your values	32
3. Curious	40
A letter to your future self	47
4. Courageous	56
Taking action	57
5. Capable	66
The Great I AM	69
6. Closed	78
Taking time out to do nothing but be	80
7. Creative	84
7-Day Creative Challenge	85
8. Connected	88
Love, value and choices	89
9. Compassionate	100
Practicing kindness and compassion	102
An exercise in self-compassion	105
10. Concordant	108
Putting it all together	108
The Final Words	112

Welcome to your *Wholeness Quest*
Workbook & Journal

Your life belongs to you.

You can choose to let it slip through your fingers, going through the motions of a partly-written version, or you can choose to live fully and consciously.

You can live a life that expresses the very best of who you are, and everything you can be.

If you're ready for that challenge, then it's time to stop searching outside for answers. It's time to look inside, and to begin the most dangerous adventure of all—the quest towards a whole new version of you.

> "Journal writing is a voyage to the interior."
>
> ~ Christina Baldwin ~

Trust your intuition. Give yourself time to listen. Use *The Wholeness Quest Workbook & Journal* to explore the signposts along your own Heroine's Journey.

Behind the 10 signposts of my *Heroine's Journey*

If you already know about my own Quest for Wholeness, you can skip this section and go on to the next, or you can read it later.

A few short years ago, despite what it looked like from the outside, (great partner, family, friends, home, and job), I most certainly did not have my life sorted.

Far from being a confident, *"I've got it all together"* woman, I felt lost, miserable, and was becoming more and more despondent. I kept asking myself, *"Is this as good as it gets?"* and alternated that with *"You have so much, stop being selfish and self-indulgent."*

I was doing everything that was expected of me. But, in reality, the version of me that was showing up was merely surviving, going through the motions of living.

I was existing behind this huge wall that I'd built to keep myself from drowning after the death, in 1997, of my young daughter Jacqueline Bree.

I finally got to the point where I had to make a change or bust. I'd tried physical changes, I completed a triathlon and ran a marathon. I tried mental changes, learning philosophy and exploring different views on the meaning of life. While all these actions brought some change, they didn't make me happy, or fill the enormous hole in my life.

I envied people who had it all together, they appeared to be so clear on their purpose, and pursued it relentlessly. These superstars confidently side-stepped procrastination and overwhelm as they trotted past me on their way to their goal. Many offered formulas that could guarantee that if you followed their process, you too could find your purpose, make a million dollars, attract a mate, lose weight, and be successful in whatever your chosen field was.

Well, call me naïve (or stupid), but when I started out on my Quest for Wholeness, I tried a few of these formulaic guru steps—okay, more than a few. (At one stage I had some friends threaten an intervention if I bought one more online course.)

While there was often some worth and many courses or workshops helped me become more conscious of my values, my priorities, and my skills—the big epiphany didn't happen. Successfully identifying my purpose, the meaning for my life, remained an illusion. In fact, I often felt worse, as if I'd failed again and was still unclear on why I was so lost.

If only I could know what I'm meant to do in this life, I could do it.

Seriously, I can get stuff done. Point me at a job and I'm like a machine. And right there is the problem. I could _think_ my way out of anything but I couldn't _feel_ deeply, I'd forgotten how.

Now, I know you can already see a flaw in me following someone else's formula to find my way. I want you to keep this in mind as _you_ work through the exercises in this workbook and journal. Each person is unique, and you are the world's expert on what's best for you. Each person's picture of success is unique to them.

It gradually dawned on me—and my bank balance—that what I was doing was not working. I had to find my own way.

I was the best person to find my purpose because I was the one who would know when it felt right, when it fit my picture of success. I wasn't all those other stars and gurus. I was me: a woman, a writer, a change agent, a coach, a leader, a mother, a wife, a sister, a lover, a friend, a reader, a runner, an introvert, etc...

So many of us seem intent on finding that one thing, that single reason for existence, that solitary purpose that means our life is worth breathing in and breathing out.

These days I don't believe it's just one thing for very many of us. The journey is the thing—the learning along your Quest for Wholeness.

My answers were not solely in other people's programs. Those programs had some of the signposts, but I couldn't follow them all the way because I needed to find my own direction, set my own destination.

My building frustration culminated in an honest conversation with a couple of friends a few years back. I admitted that despite the outward trappings of success, I was not happy. And, woohoo! Neither were they. We were all members of the *Discontented Women's Club*. We vowed to do something to get our joy back.

I began to listen more closely to an internal friend who has been with me all my life—my curiosity. I began to sit quietly and pay attention, not to anyone else, but to myself, the intuition, the inner knowing. And I began to explore.

Fast forward a few years, books, workshops, retreats, and conversations later, and I am living my remarkable life. Remarkable means worthy of attention, your attention, and you are absolutely worthy of attention.

It's time to invest in your own future.

This Wholeness Quest Workbook and Journal has some of my favourite things to suggest when people are ready to pay attention, ready to step into their driver's seat and live a remarkable life. I used these mindful reflection exercises on my own Wholeness Quest. They can help you find the signposts along your journey.

They can also deepen your reading experience of reading my memoir "*Breathing While Drowning: One Woman's Quest for Wholeness*". It isn't essential to read my book to use or find value in this workbook and journal—but it may help.

My 10 signposts were: Conflicted and Confused, Conscious, Curious, Courageous, Capable, Closed, Creative, Connected, Compassionate, and Concordant. These 10 signposts helped me to answer the question...

"How do I work out what I'm meant to be doing with my life?"

You may find that completing the exercises helps you get closer to working out what you'd like to do, and who you'd like to be. They can help you create a list of actions that will get you closer to actually living your dream and purpose. I've watched these exercises work time and again for all sorts of people, at all sorts of stages and ages of life.

One thing I know for sure. To really make change stick, we need to have 3 things happening:

1. First, our _emotional self_ needs to be persuaded to get involved and change—we need to feel it and sense it, to create the burning platform.
2. Secondly, our _logical brain_ needs to see rationally how and why we need to go there—it needs to be reasonable.
3. Finally, we need a _path_ to get there. We need the steps and the signposts to the destination—small steps, reduce stress.

The exercises under each signpost tick each of these three things. I hope they'll help you to find your own signposts and get you closer to who you want to be, and the life you want to live, fully and joyfully.

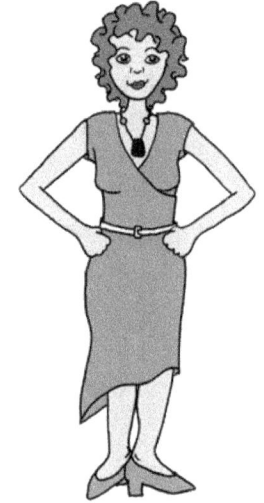

Find your dream, choose your direction, then go and do it, now!

Veronica xox

The Wholeness Quest Workbook & Journal

Start right here. Use these lines to jot down a few thoughts on what brings you to this point in your life. Why did you pick up this workbook & journal?

Where are you now? How do you feel? What are you thinking and doing?

A word on *journalling* before you begin

If you are already a journaller, or you'd rather go straight to the exercises, turn the page and go for it.

If you're anything like me, you may want to know <u>why</u> first. Why is journalling helpful? Why do I need to journal?

Here are just some of the beneficial reasons for keeping a journal.

1. An attitude of gratitude

Journalling about gratitude helps us refocus and balance some of our naturally occurring negativity. It helped me recognise the little joys in my life as well as the big ones. It reminded me to spend time celebrating what I had, rather than always thinking I needed more, or I wasn't enough. And, as I accumulated more things to be grateful for, I realised how loved I was by my family and friends.

2. Jumping for joy

Gathering those joyful moments in one place is a gift for yourself on those days when you wonder if it's all worth it. You can browse through your journal and bask in some of the fabulous, brilliant, and awesome things you've accomplished, some of the great comments from friends, family, colleagues or clients, and spend a few minutes reminding yourself how remarkable you are.

3. Practical benefits

For me, journalling almost always comes with a practical component. Recording a diary of work or family events can be a life saver. It can help you keep track of your meetings, tasks, successes, and mistakes. You can keep a journal of milestones your children have reached or funny things they've said and done. The last type of entry is very helpful when you're putting together a loving or embarrassing— or both—speech for your children's 21st birthday, graduation, or wedding.

4. Mental wellbeing benefits

Journalling can give you a safe, cathartic release for the stresses of daily life and work. It can help you feel good, recognising what you've achieved, and seeing the patterns in your life. Journalling can help you to relive events you've experienced in a safe environment where you can process them without fear or stress. Journalling regularly about both the thinking and feeling is the key.

An extra note from V.S.:

The journals I wrote to all my children are precious.

Those that I wrote to my daughter Jacqueline Bree were an incredibly important part of my healing and reconnection to life, decades after she died.

> "What a comfort is this journal I tell myself to myself, and throw the burden on my book, and feel relieved."
>
> ~ Anne Lister ~

How to use this workbook & journal

Here's what to do...

Give yourself the permission, space, and time to begin your Quest by scheduling in a few minutes each day, or an hour or two each week, to do an exercise from this journal, or to just write down your thoughts.

There will be a lot of things for you to think, feel, and write about as you follow the signposts.

So, final instructions:

- Find a pen or pencil that feels comfortable in your hand.
- Use different colour pens or the same one.
- Doodle in the margins or draw pictures all over the page.
- Stick things in or just write words.
- Let your journal get messy.

Just get it done!

Regular journalling is going to help you become more conscious of your actions, feelings, thoughts, and beliefs. You might find yourself tracking your mood and seeing patterns in your actions, such as certain people or situations that trigger certain responses in yourself. Once you've noticed them, you can choose to respond differently, or not.

No one is going to check your journal except you. It belongs to you, so there is no need for editing or correcting.

There is no right or best entry.

You can't get this wrong.

So just write anything and everything you think, feel, do, and believe.

When do I journal?

Whenever you feel like it is a good place to start. Though it's really helpful to set up your journalling as a ritual; a routine that you can repeat at the same time everyday and every week. Setting up the ritual helps you to minimise decision making and change your behaviour. It helps the change stick.

Journal every morning while you're having breakfast, or as soon as you've dropped children off at school, or jumped on the train to work, or with your first cup of tea.

Evenings are good as well, keep your journal by the bed, and jot down your thoughts about your day or your week. Evenings were my favourite. I knew that I would get to bed eventually.

You might prefer fewer times, so pick one or two days of the week when you know you'll have time to sit and think, and write. You can jot a few quick reminder notes throughout the week, and then sit down on Sunday night to journal, contemplate the week that was, and plan for the week that will be.

There is something magic in seeing your thoughts flow out on to the paper, sometimes in dribs and drabs, and sometimes in a flood.

You can start with dot points, or use a stream of consciousness.

Don't stop for grammar and literary correctness, remember no one is going to see this except you.

Begin!

> "Who you are is a necessary step to being who you will be."
>
> ~ Emmanuel ~

1. Conflicted & *confused*

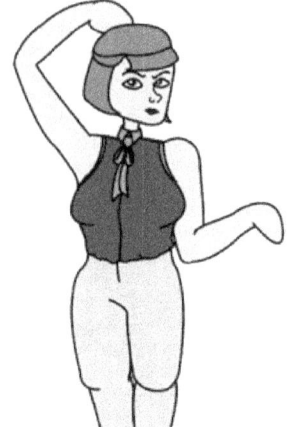

Confusion has a tendency to show up again and again—just in case you missed it the first time.

Living consciously and working on your own personal transformation is not all rainbows and roses. The moment you begin to question, conflicts arise and confusion reigns.

For me, confusion a sign that change is coming.

It can take a while to spot that you're swirling in the same spot and headed for the drain. Sometimes a gentle poke from a friend is a great reminder. Your journal is your friend.

You may have bought this workbook and journal because in some part of your life you're feeling incomplete, unfulfilled, discontent. You might be frustrated that despite an apparently good life, there is a big fat emptiness somewhere around your chest area that you just can't fill, no matter how much stuff you have or do.

Or you've made a start on finding out a little more about yourself and are still looking for more clarity, a way out of the conflict and confusion.

Being conflicted entails substantial uncertainty. It's fear that you're heading in the wrong direction, that you're going to fail, or that you're going to succeed and garner unwanted attention, or that you're going to end up alone, again.

If you've read *"Breathing While Drowning: One Woman's Quest for Wholeness"*, you've read in my story that I've had decades of conflict with myself, with others, with my work, and with the world.

All of this is okay.

The confusion is okay.

The awakening to feelings of spiritual aridity is okay.

If that's what you feel, then that's what you need to feel right now.

The growing dissatisfaction, the frustration, the hollowness.

It's all a big, fat signpost that there is something not right, and you need to find out what it is, and then DO SOMETHING ABOUT IT!

Take all the time you need to experience these feelings, let them come.

Remember, feel.

If you need to, ask for help or ask for time alone.

When you're ready, you'll reach for the next step.

This signpost is first because, for me, it was the most important one.

> *"The first step towards getting somewhere is to decide you're not going to stay where you are."*
> ~ J. P. Morgan ~

What brought you to this page? What's confusing you right now? How are you conflicted? Record your thoughts here.

_____

_____

_____

_____

_____

_____

_____

Starting a gratitude journal

Gratitude takes up space in your brain that anxiety or fear might otherwise occupy. And there's a whole lot of science that points to gratitude improving your health and wellbeing through the stimulation of the autonomic nervous system.

In short, it calms things down. And helps you remember that there are many, many things to be grateful for.

> "Piglet noticed that even though he had a Very Small Heart, it could hold rather a large amount of Gratitude."
>
> ~ A. A. Milne ~
> Winne-the-Pooh

As humans, we're wired to the negative, it takes a more conscious mindful person, to focus on the positive and to tip the balance back the other way.

Keeping a gratitude journal is a simple way to become more mindful, and to get a better handle on what is keeping you confused and conflicted.

Practising gratitude can be life changing. It certainly was for me.

Practising gratitude can increase your happiness levels by about 25%. Yep, I'd agree with that. I've read the science behind this, and I've experienced it myself—it works. There are lots of ways to practice gratitude. Journalling about it worked for me.

Here's what to do...

Start right now. Use this page to begin.

Write down 3 things you're grateful for. It can be anything big or small. Write whatever comes to mind or use the prompts on the following pages.

If you think back about your day you can often find a little something, like a flower or bird you saw, or someone who smiled at you, or the soft chair you're now sitting in. Look around you, remember your day, and find those three things.

Some days you'll have exciting things to write down.

And some days you'll be writing about very simple joys, like finding a parking spot, that first sip of a great cuppa, or a hug from a child.

There are blank pages after these instructions if you need more lines.

3 things I'm grateful for today are:

1. _____

2. _____

3. _____

Write down how you feel about those 3 things right now. The next few pages have lots more lines for your thoughts. If you run out of space, there are more lined pages in the back of this book.

If you still find it a bit difficult to get started, think about these questions:
- What's the best thing that happened today?
- Who or what inspired me today?
- What made me smile today?
- 3 things I got done today are... And I feel... about them.
- 3 things I'm going to do tomorrow are... And I feel... about them

Conflicted & Confused

30-day gratitude challenge

I recommend you write down 3 things you are grateful for daily, for 30 days. You may start to notice a change in how you view the world.

Don't worry if you miss a day, don't give up on the whole thing, just keep going when you do remember. Make it easy by putting in a trigger such as leaving your journal and a pen by your bed so you're reminded to use it before you sleep.

I found recording my gratitude easiest to do at night, it helped me remember the best parts of my day, and helped me feel good as I went off to sleep, rather than worrying about all the things I hadn't done, and would need to do tomorrow.

I have a nightly ritual to write down at least five things I'm grateful for. At the time of writing this, I'm up to entry 16,168. That's a lot to be grateful for.

If you get yourself into the habit, then you start to look forward to your 5 minutes of writing before you sleep. Sometimes, you'll find yourself during the day thinking… I'm grateful for this. I'm glad I finished that. I'm looking forward to this.

If you'd rather journal your gratitude in the morning, try thinking about your 3 things when you're drinking your first coffee or tea for the day—or while you're in the queue waiting to order. Each time you take a sip, think of something you're grateful for.

At the end of every week, give yourself some time to read back over all the entries, and think about how much you have to be grateful for in your life.

An extra note from V.S.:

One of the very first things I did on my own quest, that re-set my thoughts and changed my confused and conflicted attitude, was to start a gratitude journal. I began several years ago with a 30-day challenge and a great deal of scepticism. But it changed me! I was far happier, and amazed at how many good people, things, and moments there were in my life.

Conflicted & Confused

Day 1   *Date:*

Day 2   *Date:*

Day 3   *Date:*

Day 4   Date:

Day 5   Date:

Day 6   Date:

Conflicted & Confused

Day 7 (readback day)　　　　　　　　Date:

Day 8　　　　　　　　　　　　　　　Date:

Day 9　　　　　　　　　　　　　　　Date:

The Wholeness Quest Workbook & Journal

Day 10   *Date:*

Day 11   *Date:*

Day 12   *Date:*

Conflicted & Confused

Day 13   Date:

Day 14 (readback day)   Date:

Day 15   Date:

The Wholeness Quest Workbook & Journal

Day 16   *Date:*

Day 17   *Date:*

Day 18   *Date:*

Conflicted & Confused

Day 19　　　　　　　　　　　　　　　　　　Date:

Day 20　　　　　　　　　　　　　　　　　　Date:

Day 21 (readback day)　　　　　　　　　　　Date:

Day 22   Date:

Day 23   Date:

Day 24   Date:

Conflicted & Confused

Day 25   *Date:*

Day 26   *Date:*

Day 27   *Date:*

Day 28 (readback day) Date:

Day 29 Date:

Day 30 Date:

Time to do a final read back.

Remember, keeping a gratitude journal is a simple way to become more mindful, and to get a better handle on what is keeping you confused and conflicted.

Are there any themes or patterns in what you're grateful for? Does that suggest anything to you?

How did you feel after you'd read back over 30 days of gratitude? There are some lined pages overleaf to record your thoughts.

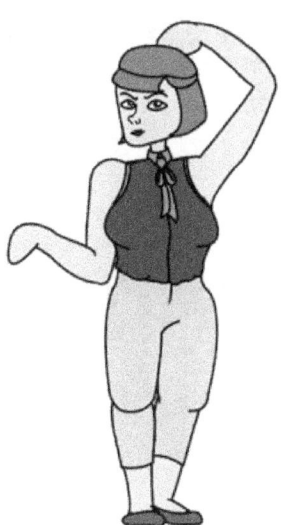

Don't stop here. Keep recording your gratitude either daily or once a week. Use the back of this journal or get yourself a blank book just for gratitude and get writing.

When you're ready, move on to the second signpost – don't leave it too long.

Schedule some time in your diary now.

"The miracle of gratitude is that is shifts your perception to such an extent, that it changes the world you see."

~ Dr Robert Holden ~

Conflicted & Confused

2. Conscious

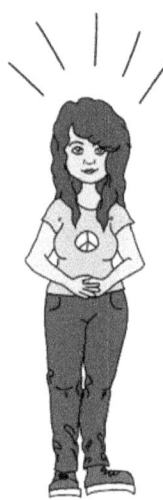

The next signpost is about becoming more conscious, waking up from the deep sleep of quiet desperation, loss, frustration, apathy, monotony, or other dissatisfaction in your life. Waking up to the awareness of who you are. Realising your separation from your life lived fully and joyfully.

It's always been somewhere over there, outside of you. Now you begin to realise that the dissatisfaction is anchored inside. The conflicted and confused starts to seek a greater awareness.

You are the sum of all your choices and experiences up to this point in your life.

You're ready, willing, and committed to change. At this signpost, you grow your awareness of who you are now, and what you bring to your life.

Build on what you're grateful for from signpost 1. Reflect on your strengths, your values, and the things that are important in your life—your big reasons why. Why do you want to change? Who do you want to become? What do you want to do? People who are conscious of who they are, and what their strengths and values are, enjoy happier, healthier, more productive, and more purposeful lives.

There are a million ways you can get more conscious about what's important. Just by thinking and reading you become more aware. The best way I found to start was to journal—of course. Start regularly writing down what you're thinking, feeling, and doing. Do this every day at the same time, you can follow on from your gratitude list, or start a separate journal if you prefer.

Remember to make it easy to do by leaving your journal and pen beside the bed, and write just before you go to sleep or first thing when you wake in the morning.

If you're not used to journalling, give yourself a question or two to answer:

When was my happiest moment today?

What was I thinking, doing, and feeling today?

And then go a little deeper.

What do I believe? What are the things I value? Why?

Am I being true to my values in how I work and play and live?

What are my strengths?

What makes me successful at what I do?

If you're not sure of your strengths, think about the things that you can do effortlessly, the things that you love to do, that energise you.

If you'd like to discover more about your strengths both realised and unrealised, go to my True Dialogue website (https://truedialogue.com.au/leadership-coaching/work-with-a-coach/) and book an Expert Strengths Profile assessment and debrief.

> "Be a first-rate version of yourself, instead of a second-rate version of somebody else."
>
> ~ Judy Garland ~

Exploring your values

What's important to me?

Your values feed what's important to you in life. They're part of your big "why".

Knowing your values helps you understand what drives you to get up in the morning and do it all again—what you enjoy, what inspires you and what you'd like more of in your life. Becoming aware of what's important to you is a great step towards living more consciously and confidently.

By building a life and lifestyle around your values, you create a life that's more meaningful to you, and one which expresses the very best of who you are.

Your values may change over time as you gather experience and deepen as you understand yourself better. Your values can also be situational, so what's true for you at work may not be as important at home and vice versa.

The values listed here are only to give you some ideas, there may be other words you'll want to add that better capture what's important to you.

Remember: When it comes to **values**, there's no right or wrong—only who **you** are!

Do this exercise once or twice a year, at least. It helps you reconnect to what's important.

Here's what to do…

First...

- Grab a pen and find a quiet spot.
- Close your eyes. Take 3 long, slow, deep breaths. Now breathe away normally.
- Open your eyes and without over thinking it, let your eyes and hand run down the lines and underline any word in the list that feels important to you. If you feel like a word is missing, or one pops into your head, add it to the list.

Conscious

Abundance	Duty	Ingenuity	Responsibility
Acceptance	Ease	Innovation	Resourcefulness
Accomplishment	Economic security	Integrity	Romance
Accuracy	Efficiency	Intellectual status	Safety
Acknowledgement	Effortlessness	Intimacy	Security
Achievement	Empowerment	Inspiration	Self-esteem
Adventure	Energy	Intuition	Self-reliance
Affection	Enthusiasm	Justice	Self-respect
Ambition	Expertise	Joy	Sensuality
Arts	Environment	Kindness	Service to others
Authenticity	Excellence	Knowledge	Service to society
Autonomy	Fairness	Leadership	Silence
Balance	Fame	Learning	Silliness
Beauty	Family & friends	Listening	Simplicity
Boldness	Flexibility	Love	Sophistication
Calmness	Ethical practice	Loyalty	Spirituality
Capability	Fearlessness	Meaning	Spontaneity
Challenge	Fitness	Mindfulness	Stability
Change	Frankness	Money	Status
Clarity	Focus	Nature	Stillness
Collaboration	Forgiveness	Obedience	Strength
Community	Freedom	Optimism	Success
Compassion	Friendship	Orderliness	Tact
Concern for others	Fun	Participation	Teamwork
Confidence	Generosity	Partnership	Thankfulness
Connectedness	Gentleness	Passion	Thoughtfulness
Contentment	Groundedness	Patience	Tolerance
Communication	Growth	Peace	Tradition
Compassion	Happiness	Personal growth	Tranquillity
Consciousness	Hard work	Practicality	Travel
Contentment	Harmony	Presence	Trust
Contribution	Having a family	Pride	Truth
Cooperation	Health	Productivity	Usefulness
Courage	Helpfulness	Prosperity	Understanding
Creativity	Hopefulness	Purpose	Unity
Curiosity	Honesty	Reason	Variety
Determination	Honour	Recognition	Vision
Directness	Humour	Relaxation	Vitality
Discovery	Idealism	Reflection	Wealth
Diversity	Impact	Resilience	Willingness
Dreaming	Independence	Respect	Wisdom

33

The Wholeness Quest Workbook & Journal

Second...

- Look at all the words you've underlined and choose your top 5 values
- Write the top 5 down here and add a few words about why they feel important to you right at this moment.

Don't overthink it, just write whatever pops into your mind.

Value 1 is   *and this is how I feel about it...*

Value 2 is   *and this is how I feel about it...*

Value 3 is _____ and this is how I feel about it…

Value 4 is _____ and this is how I feel about it…

Value 5 is _____ and this is how I feel about it…

Third...

- Choose your number one value—the one that stands out the most. What's *the* word that sits at the core of you and your life right now?
- Write about how this value relates to your past decisions?
- Write about one decision that this value may have influenced in your work or home life.

My number 1 value right now is...

This value and its relationship to my past decisions...

A decision this value may have influenced in my work or home life…

Fourth, and finally…

- Now that you're beginning to work out what's important to you—what are you going to do with that information?

- Start by writing down one area of your life where you're going to use what you value to make different choices. If could be at work, with family and friends, or on your leisure time.

- Make it easy on yourself. Pick one area and one action, try if for a few days.

- Spend five minutes each evening before you go to sleep writing about any moments in the day when you did or thought or felt something connected to that value.

- After you've written, do a check-in. Does it still feel as though this is your number 1 value at the moment?

So far, if you're keeping up your gratitude exercise as well, you're journalling about gratitude, how you're feeling, your value, and any random thoughts or insights.

An extra note from V.S.:

Doing this exercise annually helps keep me connected to my why. Some of my values always stay the same, and often different ones move up the priority scale depending on what I'm doing in my personal and professional life.

> "Whether you're keeping a journal or writing as a meditation,
> it's the same thing.
> What's important is you're having a relationship with your mind."
>
> ~ Natalie Goldberg ~

This is the area of my life and the action I'm going to take by using my number 1 value to make different choices.

3. Curious

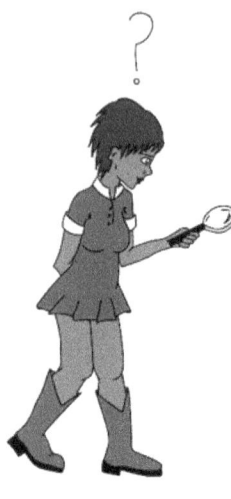

Curiosity is the next signpost.

What could I do, where could I go, who could I be? What does it all mean—life, the universe and everything?

Start thinking about the possibilities of becoming the person you want to be, and exploring and experiencing what you have to do to get there.

It's time to dust off all those childhood dreams and give them another chance. It's never too late to start again.

If you don't build your dream, someone will hire you to help build theirs.
~Tony Gaskins~

The first time I saw this Tony Gaskins quote, I had a big AHA. I realised that I'd been working on other people's dreams for decades. It was definitely time to start working on my own.

Now that you're remembering what you value and what's important to you, who you want to be, and maybe even a hint of what you want to do, it's time to write yourself a plan for getting there.

This step is also about getting organised and back on track, creating strategies that can give you step-by-step actions to get to where you want to go.

Stretching your curiosity

I often use my Six Faithful Friends to frame my curiosity questions.

I have six faithful friends, they taught me all I knew...

Their names are why and what and when and where and how and who!

Here's what to do...

Try the questions below to get you started using some of my six faithful friends... You may think of others once your curiosity is piqued. There are extra pages at the back of the journal if you run out of space here.

Write down anything that comes up when you ask yourself:

- Why do I feel like I do right now? How do I want to feel? Why is how I feel important?

≈ Who would I be if I could be anyone I want? What is it that I really desire?

"Imagination is the beginning of creation. You imagine what you desire, you will what you imagine, and at last, you create what you will."

~ George Bernard Shaw ~

❧ How can I use my strengths and what I value to live a life that expresses the very best of who I am?

∾ What have I done successfully in the past? How did I do it?

- How have other people changed their lives, started a business, or made a successful career transition? Do I need anyone to help me?

> "Curiosity only does one thing, and that is to give. And what is gives you are clues on the incredible scavenger hunt of your life."
>
> ~ Elizabeth Gilbert ~

◈ What is it that I could do right now, in my life, at my workplace, or in my relationships to change how I am being?

"Curiosity is the beginning of wisdom."

~ Françoise Sagan ~

A letter to your future self

Think of your dream life as if it were a long-awaited holiday. If you were going on a holiday, would you just get in the car and start driving without a destination?

Where would you go?

What would you take with you?

How would you know if you were heading in the right direction, or when you had arrived?

How would you make sure there was some FUN happening along the way, or ADVENTURE or THRILLS—or whatever floats your boat?

This exercise builds on the previous two. Now that you've got a bit of a sense of what's important to you from starting the gratitude journal and doing the values exercise, it's time to start putting words to your dream and your purpose.

> "Never forget: this very moment we can change our lives.
> There was never a moment, and there never will be,
> where we are without the power to alter our destiny"
> ~ Steven Pressfield ~

Here's what to do...

Choose a date some months or even years ahead that means something to you. An anniversary or a birthday works well.

Find a quiet place to sit, give yourself at least half an hour, turn to a blank page in your journal and make sure you have your favourite pen.

- Close your eyes for a few moments and imagining that a miracle has happened.

Your life has turned out exactly the way you wanted it to.

- Imagine how you would feel if you were living the life of your dreams, a life full of meaning and joy, success and purpose.

- Now, write a letter telling yourself about everything that's happening in your life. Describe your perfect day in as much detail and colour as you can:

    - Describe sights, sounds, tastes, include how you feel, what you're doing, where you are, and who's with you.

    - Look in your future diary and see what you've got planned for the day, the week, the year – work or pleasure or a mix of both.

    - Imagine checking your bank balance and watching the income pouring in.

    - Where are you off to work, look around at your workspace. Or are you working from home or part-time or online? Or are you retired and finished work for good?

    - Are you volunteering somewhere? Or mentoring the next generation?

    - Who are you having lunch with? Can you taste what's on the menu?

    - Who are you playing with?

    - Listen, what can you hear? Music, laughter, conversations, quiet?

    - What can you smell? Food, fragrance, fresh air?

    - See yourself opening your wardrobe and trying out your new clothes. Feel the material, the textures against your skin.

Whatever looks, sounds, smells and feels right – this is your dream.

Write until you feel finished.

How do you feel?

Enjoy, and be curious about what you discover.

Start your letter over the page...

An extra note from V.S.:

I wrote my first letter to my future self on Saturday 14th September 2013, and it was an amazingly liberating experience. It gave me some curious revelations. Many of the things I wrote about have become reality, and others are well on the way.

If you want to read the full letter, it's on page 362 of "Breathing While Drowning".

> "Ask for what you want, and be prepared to get it."
>
> ~ Maya Angelou ~

The Wholeness Quest Workbook & Journal

Dear Future Me,   *Date:*

Curious

Curious

Let yourself dream, it doesn't cost anything to dream.

Now that you have a dream destination in mind, how can you put your dreams out into the world?

Sometimes writing your letter will prompt you to remember or to realise what your dreams are. The next signpost will help you to take action on your letter, but, you can start right now.

Here's what to do...

To help you picture your dream destination more clearly, pick one of the activities below and make a start on adding some life and colour into your dreams.

- Make a dream board, cut out or draw pictures of your dreams and stick the board somewhere that you'll see it every day, and give yourself time to look

- Write, draw, or doodle your dreams—and then put them on that dream board

- Talk to someone you trust, tell them what you're thinking and dreaming about—read them your letter

Need some more help to shape your dreams?

- Subscribe to blogs by people who you admire or whose message feels like it has something to say to you.

- Go to a workshop or three

- Read a book or six

- Get a coach or a mentor, someone who can be your confidential thinking partner, someone who'll be in your corner, ferociously focused on you, and keeping you on track.

4. Courageous

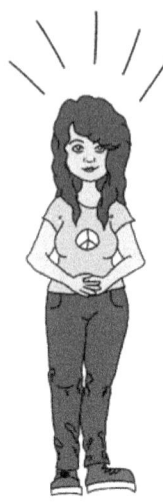

The next signpost is courage.

Leap into the darkness, try stuff, think differently, think deeply. This is the road of trials, so be warned, it might involve meeting ogres and dragons.

I sometimes wondered for myself if maybe it's not courage, so much as a lack of fear, or sensible precaution talking. Some would say acting without fear is reckless, impulsive, or impetuous.

For me, sometimes it felt like the word was desperate. But no, adventurous is how I'm living my life, and my life is my own personal adventure!

> *"Courage is contagious.*
> *Every time we choose courage,*
> *we make everyone around us a little better and the world a little braver."*
> *~ Brené Brown ~*

How about you?

It's time to build on what you've thought about who you want to be, and what you want to do, it's time for you to get courageous.

This step is about taking real action, small or large, to do something different. But it's not just any old action—although even that will help. This is action with a strategic intent.

And action in the right direction *is* traction—remember the plan, the goal, the dream.

Do something different, and do it now… don't wait until it's perfect.

Progress trumps perfection every time.

Taking action

If you keep in mind your values, your strengths, and your dreams; the actions just about line up and do themselves—just about.

You still need to take that first step, and there are some days that it will be a grind.

The only way out is through.

You may be amazed how coincidences and serendipity seem to ramp up as soon as you commit to action.

Intent is good. Action is better. Doing both together is best.

Did you know?

80% of people don't set goals…

Of the **20%** who do set goals…

16% think of their goals but don't write them down…

4% write them down but don't regularly review them…

Only **1%** actually write them down and regularly review them.

Those **1%** of people are in the top achievers in the world.
(Thanks for those figures Leonie Dawson www.leoniedawson.com).

How easy is that!

Just by thinking of your dream goals, writing them down and regularly reviewing them you can change your life.

> "You have BRAINS in your HEAD.
> You have FEET in your SHOES.
> You can STEER yourself in any DIRECTION you CHOOSE."
> ~ Dr Suess~

> *"A goal is a dream with a deadline."*
> *~ Napoleon Hill ~*

You can set a goal and it can stay a dream if you don't do anything about it.

Your commitment has the power to make goals—and dreams come true.

Achieving your goal can sometimes depend on other people or things not totally under your control. Commitments, however, what you take action to do yourself, are totally within your control.

An extra note from V.S.:

Writing and publishing a book was my dream. It stayed a dream until I was ready to commit to action.

I set a smaller goal of writing at least 300 words a day and I made a commitment to get up at 5:30 every morning to write.

External accountability was also important for me. I joined a Facebook Group as my external accountability partners. They helped me with early morning write-ins and lots of encouragement. Now, I'm part of the #6amAusWriters group on Twitter who encourage each other every morning.

It took me about 7 months to get my first book done, and some days I wrote more than others, but eventually I got to the final 116,555 words. Breathing While Drowning was ready to publish.

Sounds so easy when you write it like that. There were plenty of ups and downs, but it was the commitment that got me to my goal and my dream.

Here's what to do...

Step 1

Go back to your *letter to your future self*. With a highlighter, mark the big signposts that come up in the story, the things that will have to change to move you from where you are and who you are now. This could be a new skill you now have, a new job, a new home, a new relationship, a new way of thinking or feeling or being.

Take one long slow deep breath, choose one signpost you want to start with, if this feels too big, pick a smaller one and start with that.

Here's an example

You may have written that you *"are relaxed and calm at work and spend time regularly practicing meditation"*. What are the steps you need to get there?

As you make the first task, try to imagine the very first action you could take that would get you started.

- Schedule meditation into the calendar (Hang on a minute I don't know how to meditate!)

- Learn meditation (How am I going to learn ? Remember my values and how I prefer to learn)

- Book into a course on meditation (Do I know of any good courses near me?)

- Google meditation courses near me (What if I don't have any extra funds?)

- Check YouTube for meditation videos or download a free meditation app onto phone (try the Healthy Minds Program from the Center for Healthy Minds—University of Wisconsin)

- Schedule 5-min meditation into calendar four times a day – HOORAH!

So, the very first thing you might do to reach your goal of being—*"relaxed and calm at work and spend time regularly practicing meditation"*—is head to YouTube and search for meditation videos or your app store to download one that looks and sounds right onto your phone.

Now it's your turn

Ready to pick your first milestone? Do it now.

What are the main actions you'll need to take to reach that first milestone? Will you need things or people to help you get the action done?

Step 2

Next, transfer those actions to the Dream Action Plan layout on the next page and pick a time to get each action done by, write this down too, use colours and big print. If you like pictures, paste these with your words.

You may prefer to create the Dream Action Plan on a separate larger sheet and put it up on the wall where you can see it everyday.

Step 3

Finally, tell a good friend about your dream and goals and ask them to keep you accountable for the getting the actions done. If they don't want to, maybe you can find someone else who will support you.

Look around you. Jim Rohn famously suggested...

"You are the average of the five people you spend the most time with."

Are the people you're spending the most time with helping you grow or holding you back? Do they want to come with you and grow too, or are they frightened that your light will shine on their darkness? Maybe it's time to let some people go, and open up to others.

Step 4

All that's left is to take action and keep taking action, ticking off the tasks and steps. And when you've finished one list, go back to your letter and pick up the next goal.

Reflect, re-plan, and repeat.

Journal about the things you've done and what you've learnt about yourself, your path, and your purpose.

Don't forget to go back to the dream regularly to check you're still heading in the right direction. Once you've got your first few small actions under your belt, check on your dream goals. *Reflect* on how you felt getting stuff done—or not, what worked and what didn't. *Re-plan* if you need to, then repeat the small action steps. *Repeat* as often as you need to get to your dreams.

"Success is the sum of small efforts, repeated day-in and day-out."
~ Robert Collier ~

Dream Action Plan

Action	Things and people I need to help me get it done	I will complete this by Date:	Done? Yes or No

Courageous

The Wholeness Quest Workbook & Journal

Dream Action Plan

Action	Things and people I need to help me get it done	I will complete this by Date:	Done? Yes or No

Courageous

5. Capable

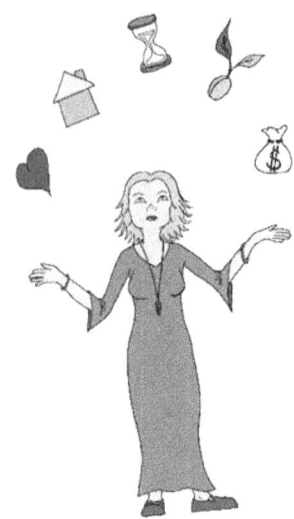

The next signpost is about being capable and finding your own competence, not the illusory boon of success.

This is not just about: job, position, responsibility, homes, holidays, and so forth. It's about whatever it takes to make you feel like you are competently making your difference in the world.

I prefer the word capable to competence, because capable feels so much more optimistic and *enabling* in my mind.

Now I realise my capabilities, and I use them to be who I want to be, to work with people I love, and to create programmes that free people to explore their own potential to be themselves. And if I don't know something, I find someone who does, and learn from them.

This step is about realising you can do things differently and building your own capability and agility. It's about finding your zone of genius. It's about checking your commitment to growth.

Being capable is being able to achieve, either efficiently and effectively or kind of just getting there, regardless of what you want to do.

This step is also about practising, lots of practising, and experiencing what it takes to be the best you that you can be.

> *"The only person you are destined to become is the person you decide to be."*
> *~ Ralph Waldo Emerson ~*

Think about driving a car. When you first learn, you have to concentrate on every little thing. After a few years, you do many of the things automatically and can talk and drive at the same time. It's important to remember that action works in the present, not the future—so act now!

This step is not about judging in terms of good or bad, right or wrong; rather, it's about evaluating and analysing so you have evidence to decide.

Analysing is examining methodically to explain or interpret. This is a good reason to keep journalling.

Think about the human body ... it's amazing. Most of us don't need to remember how to breathe, it's handled automatically, but we can increase our lung capacity to get fitter or be a better speaker or singer by practising.

The brain has a huge capacity to learn and do stuff. The soul can learn even more if you give it a chance to practise.

Go back to that friend who's been keeping you accountable and ask them to help you think about stuff you are capable of doing now.

What kind of skills do you use when you're successful at things, especially the things that bring you joy? Just keep in mind when you chat to your friend that you are looking for support, not advice.

> "Surround yourself with the dreamers and the doers, the believers and thinkers, but most of all, surround yourself with those who see the greatness within you, even when you don't see it yourself."
> ~ Edmund Lee ~

Now just get on and do stuff.

By taking action, you get experience, and every experience, no matter how it feels or how it ends up, gives you more information to help you make a decision about the next step you need to take. This builds your confidence, and away you go again.

And, of course, journal it. You can get great insights into how you work, your capabilities, and innate talents by recording your thoughts when you are in the zone of genius. Then, when things are a hard slog in the future, you can choose to make different choices.

Because that's what it's all about—doing things differently.

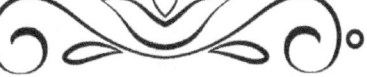

Remember this definition of stupidity…

"…doing the same thing over and over again but expecting different results."
~Albert Einstein~

To look for your zone of genius, think about what lights you up?

Ask for feedback—it's scary, but it's worthwhile. Ask someone else what they see that you're capable of. What they notice when you're doing something that lights you up or what's missing when you're dragging your heels.

It could help you to figure out what else you need to learn. And then you can go and learn it.

What does light you up? Jot down your thoughts below.

The Great I AM

This an excellent way to declare **who** you are and **why** your work matters.

No one on earth can do what you do, in precisely the way that YOU do it.

Most of us are not great at being proud and out loud about why we are awesome or brilliant or fabulous. This is your chance to have a little practice at changing that, getting your capabilities—and more on the page.

This exercise is adapted with permission from a worksheet generously shared by Alexandra Franzen, so please go and check out her website and look at all her other fabulous offerings at www.AlexandraFranzen.com

Here's what to do...

Only one rule: **Don't over think it!**

The worksheet is designed to be completed by hand on paper and FAST!

So, grab your favourite pen. Don't edit or go back and change anything, just let the thoughts jump onto the page.

The great I AM worksheet includes 10 elements.

Give yourself **TWO MINUTES** to complete each element. That's it. Set the timer.

We often give ourselves (way) too much time to make it "perfect" and send ourselves into maddening spirals of confusion in the process.

An extra note from V.S.: The first time I did this exercise, I found it really challenging, it was so hard to keep my head out of the picture and let my soul have fun. I took myself way too seriously.

When you give yourself a ferocious time limit to pour out your thoughts… magic transpires. We need to stop writing from the head and start writing from the heart and gut. As Alexandra Franzen calls it—the HUT.

So, take a deep breath, get your HUT fired up, pick up your pen, and let's go!

I am a…

Insert your job title in the box below. Don't worry if it sounds 'boring'. Don't worry if it sounds 'braggy'. Definitely don't worry if it sounds 'wacky'. Jot down the very thing that comes to your mind first.

But really, I'm a…

Who & what are you…really? What's your secret name? Your dream title? Your superhero alias? (Don't mull over it. Just go.)

Capable

I'm amazing at...

Jot down the first three or four things that bubble up, don't think too hard.

Circle the one that feels like something you'd like to be *known* for.

And I've devoted most of my life to...

Studying / exploring / questioning / mastering / helping / teaching / fixing / leading / sharing / serving / doing ... *what?*

When you work with me, you can expect...

Jot down the **benefits** that other humans receive, when they partner with you or listen to your words, or see your work, or get one of your legendary appreciations...

And you'll probably be surprised and delighted by...

Got quirks, hidden talents, or an unexpected approach to your line of work? Put it all down here.

Capable

My work matters because...

It alleviates the suffering caused by ....

Or, It makes the world a .... place

Or, It allows people to experience ....

Or, Without it, we'd all be ....

Or, what?

And I'm here to remind you that ...

This is your message, your final battle cry, the big WHY.

Here's where you get to express your values, the words that are going to be inscribed on your tombstone.

You're not confused.

You've got this!

GO.

My question for you is...

What do you secretly wonder about everyone you meet?

What do you wish your fellow human beings would ask themselves?

What's your favourite icebreaker, soul-shaker, conversation-maker?

To sum it up? I am...

...not for the faint of heart.

...the slightly-psychic aunty you always wanted, but never had.

...a work in progress.

...a work of art.

...a teacher, a student, and everything in between.

...completely astonishing.

...(your closing thought, here)

Now take a deep breath and weave it all together

You're done.

You're amazing, awesome, brilliant and fabulous. So write it down.

I am a ...

But really, I'm a ...

I'm amazing at ...

And I've devoted most of my life to ...

When you work with me, you can expect ...

And you'll probably be surprised & delighted by ...

My work matters because ...

And I'm here to remind you that …

My question for you is …

To sum it up? I am …

And you're very, very CAPABLE.

Your final challenge is to read the last section—the summary—**aloud** to someone who knows and loves you.

I dare you.

> *"Our deepest fear is not that we are inadequate.*
> *Our deepest fear is that we are powerful beyond measure.*
> *It is our light, not our darkness, that most frightens us."*
> *~ Marianne Williamson ~*

6. Closed

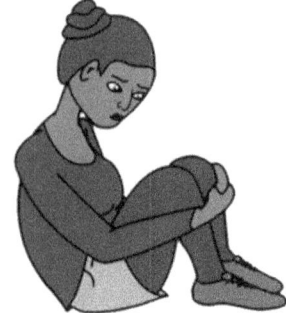

Signpost six is the initiation and descent to the goddess, death and darkness and silence. Closed.

This closed feeling can be a little scary. I found things dissipate and dissolve better if I let myself experience them. It's okay to go there.

It's okay for time alone to just be.

Closed can feel empty, waiting, lost, endless cycles of introspection, anger, sadness, diving deep into the darkness and staying there, being held, being whole.

Taking time to listen to your soul. And…

Days and weeks and months and years of being closed are like strings of dark pearls holding you together — sometimes just barely.

And then, deep in the darkness, there is comfort and time to heal and think and feel. Time to re-charge and regenerate until you're ready to show up, and step up again.

Slowly emerging, a trigger releases, realising there is something else, stepping into one of the other stages when you're ready.

Often that next stage is heralded by a burst of creativity, a new idea is born.

It entails taking off the cloak, opening to possibility, taking a breath, and living and loving again.

We can do this: be closed, and drowning, and still breathing and living.

An extra note from V.S.:

I spent a long time closed. And I keep going back whenever I need to.

After my daughter, Jacqui Bree died when she was 4-years old, I fell into an ocean of grief,

I felt like I was drowning.

It was all I could do to keep breathing, taking it moment by moment.

People kept trying to drag me out before I was ready.

I needed more time.

It took me almost 20 years to be ready, and when I was ready, the message appeared, and I opened that flood gate again.

So, you take your own sweet time.

You don't always have to be out there being what everybody else expects you to be.

Spend some time being what you want to be, on your own terms.

> "Put your ear down close to your soul, and listen hard."
> ~ Anne Sexton ~

Taking time out to do nothing but be

Taking time out can look like a whole lot of things, and I've included a few that will take just a little while. You may need a much longer time.

And there may be times when you need to reach out to professional support to help you navigate your way safely.

Here are some starters to get you into the habit of taking time out to do nothing but be.

A walk

A sit in the sun

Reading

A holiday on your own

A retreat in the bush.

Doing nothing at all.

One of the best ways I've found for getting into just being is mindfulness (meditation).

Now, even after practising mindfulness for some time, I am far from an expert.

A practice that I love as an introduction to mindfulness is the Stillness Exercise which can done sitting in a chair.

You can read the Stillness Exercise, and record yourself saying it so you can play it over and over. Or you can download me reading the Stillness Exercise from SoundCloud. (www.soundcloud.com/veronica-strachan/stillness-exercise) Eventually, you won't need to hear the words to help yourself be still.

If you decide to do the Stillness Exercise, do it every day, ideally two or three times each day to begin. This will give you time out.

Just be.

My favourite time is first thing in the morning and last thing at night. No one else is up, the house is quiet, and I can start my day closed and quiet. The stillness helps me re-charge and be ready for whatever the day has to hold.

Sometimes after your time out, you'll feel the need to write, so keep your journal handy. And if you don't, then don't.

Spend a little time researching mindfulness for yourself. Chase down some of the eastern practices which have been around for thousands of years.

Even one long, slow, deep breath can make all the difference, to taking time out. Try that now. One long, slow, deep breath—see…

The Stillness Exercise

The Stillness Exercise is a simple practice which is very old, and helps in gaining the ability to become truly still. This ability to become truly still helps to bring about a greater depth of experience, and so the stillness that is sought is not just stillness at a physical level, but it's also a stillness of the heart and mind.

Here's what to do…

Find a place where you will be uninterrupted and sit in comfortable position. A chair is fine.

Close your eyes, take one slow deep breath…

If at any point you need to open your eyes or change your position, do so—then close your eyes again, and resume the Stillness Exercise.

First, let the mind be free of any concern or preoccupation…

Let the mind fall still and come to rest within…

Be aware of where you are now…

Feel the touch of your feet on the ground...

The weight of your body on the chair...

Feel the touch of your clothes on your skin...

And the play of air on your face and hands...

If they are open, let your eyes receive colour and form without any comment...

Taste...

Smell...

Be fully here...

Now be aware of hearing...

Let sounds be received, and let them rise and fall without comment or judgment of any kind...

With your body completely relaxed, let your hearing run right out to the furthest and gentlest sounds, embracing all...

Simply rest in this great awareness for a few moments...

Stay as long as you need and when you are ready, gently bring your awareness back to your body, be present, be home.

Again, if you prefer, you can find and download a free recording of me reading the Stillness Exercise at SoundCloud (www.soundcloud.com/veronica-strachan/stillness-exercise).

> "Any activity done mindfully is a form of meditation."
> ~ Anonymous ~

How do you feel after the exercise? What thoughts came—and went—for you? Write down your thoughts below. Did you enjoy it enough to make it a habit?

7. Creative

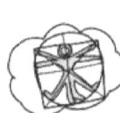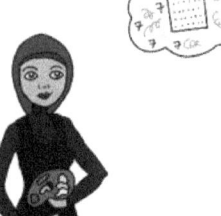

Signpost seven is creative.

For me this was part of my urgent yearning to connect with the feminine, my source of creativity. Hooray for that!

I found women who held out their hands, their arms, and their love to welcome me despite all my faults, failings, and foibles.

Get yourself into a circle of women, let them nurture you and help you hold responsibility for growing.

There are a million ways to get creative. Use your curiosity muscle and get looking and thinking about how you want to be creative.

It's time to start adding to your repertoire, putting your own mark on your life, trying more and more things, filling your life with moments of bliss and the zone of genius.

"Creativity is contagious, pass it on."
~ Albert Einstein

Keeping some things and discarding others allows you to make your life your way. Take some time to relax; creativity generally doesn't like to be forced—I know, I've tried! It prefers to sneak in when you're not concentrating, when you're least expecting it, like in the shower! Keep a notebook handy! I've often wished for a small waterproof whiteboard.

Try something different; take a risk. Get out that bucket list and start on some of those crazy ideas. Nurture your innate talent, whether it's writing, speaking, drawing, paper folding, crochet, coding, listening, golf, building, or something else.

Set aside time. You've learned by now that if it isn't on the schedule, it generally doesn't get done. So, schedule in some regular creative time.

Go to a museum, or a library, or a lake, or a magnificent building, or a dark laneway, or a festival.

Find other people who are doing what you want to do and follow their every move on social media, in the nicest possible way—no stalking, please. Then ask them for a few minutes of their time. Ask them how they get creative, and look at lining up all the parts of your life to explore that way.

One of my favourite paths to creativity—apart from writing of course—is baking. I love creating muffins, scones, cakes, slices, biscuits, desserts of all sorts. And they have the added benefit of being able to consume them, yum. Then you start all over again.

7-Day Creative Challenge

A little challenge can be good to get you started.

I took a 5-day creative challenge a few years ago, and had a whole lot of fun in 5 minutes a day. So now it's your turn. And yes, this is for 7-days because I know you have at least 2 more days in you by now.

> "You can't use up creativity.
> The more you use it, the more you have."
> ~ Maya Angelou ~

7 X 7 = 49 minutes of your week spent in creativity.

How hard could it be? How much fun could it be? Making it a challenge gives you added accountability.

Here's what to do...

1. Pick a creative activity that you love or that you'd like to try.
   If you spend a lot of time creating in one particular way or through one medium, try something different – mix it up. Anything goes!

2. Tell a friend or family member about your challenge and see if they'll get involved too. It could be a whole lot of fun if you get the whole family or a group at work engaged. If you'd rather work alone, just tell your friend you'd like to show them your stuff at the end of the 7 days. Ask them to remind you of your promise. Or add some extra accountability and post your efforts on your favourite social media platform.

3. Spend at least 7 minutes on your creative efforts every day for the next 7 days. Of course, you may like to do more than 7...

4. Journal about your creative time each day. How can you put your unique mark on all aspects of your life with this creative flavour?

Now go forth and create...

Here's some space to jot down your ideas of how to be creative...

Remember... creativity often starts with something fun.

In case nothing pops into your mind, here are some creative sparks to get you started. Or, if you have children around you, ask them what to do.

> *"Creativity is intelligence having fun."*
> ~ Albert Einstein ~

Listen to music	Knit	Write by hand (works for me)
Play music	Crochet	Daydream
Draw	Whittle	Look at something green or blue
Doodle in the pages of this workbook	Play a video game (if this is new for you)	Sit outside a box
Meditate (there it is again)	Decorate a stone	Gesture with two hands (for 7 mins remember)
Get someone else's opinion on something	Dance	Lie down and look at the sky (or the ceiling)
Go outside	Bake (OK, this may take you more than 7 minutes unless you do a raw protein ball)	Open a dictionary and find a word that's new for you. Make sentences and a story about the word.
Dig in the garden		
Think about something far away	Paint something even if it's painting concrete with water	
Make a list of unusual objects	Go for a walk	Do some yoga
	Create a secret code	Do some origami paper folding or make a paper plane (you'll need 7 different styles)
Build something (use Lego blocks or Play-Doh or Blu-Tac, or sticks and stones)	Sit in a coffee shop and make up new names for all the people you see	
		Take your favourite photos and quotes, put them together and post them on social media
Rearrange your furniture	Weave a basket	
Go to the library and flick through the art, craft, gardening or a section you wouldn't normally go to	Laugh a little, just start laughing at nothing and see what happens if you keep it up for 7 minutes	Create a treasure chest (photos, quotations etc...)

8. Connected

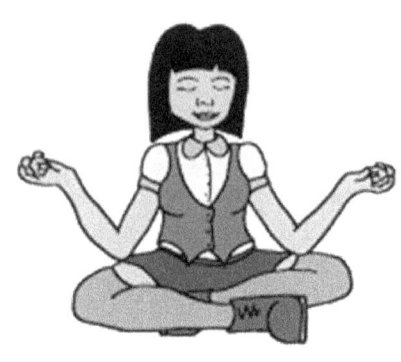

Signpost eight is get connected.

Finding some things that connect you, and ways of being that resonate.

- Connect to the light and the shadow, reconnect all the lost parts of yourself.
- Connect with your spouse, partner and children, or connect with people who are also searching.
- Connect with your purpose, your values, your dreams.

It's at this point that you begin to realise all your joy, all your success — is intimately based on how you build and interact in relationships with yourself and others.

An extra note from V.S.:

For me, being connected is celebrating who I am. It entails being vulnerable and showing up real, flawed, and fabulous, all of me. Scary at times, and it takes a while, but it's so much easier to be the real me, rather than to be someone else's version of me.

At our most basic level, we're all energy. And there is attraction and repulsion going on all the time as we live and love. When I read Anita Moorjani's words in her book 'Dying to be me' about us being all one across time and space and dimensions, it made so much sense.

Life's not either or — it's everything.

Let me explain a bit further. Getting connected is making the steps to be what you value, to live with your joys and strengths, to practise what you preach, if you like.

You've got conscious (aware of what's important to you), curious (wondering how your life can look and feel), courageous (taking the first step and realising you're capable of this and so much more), creative (you've unleashed your gifts and imagination to make your own mark), and now you're connecting (making all the dots line up to *your* specifications—for yourself, your purpose, your life).

You coordinate, consolidate, and allow all the thinking and feeling, so that you're showing up with certainty, confidence, and the willingness to act in the direction of your dreams.

> "We cannot live only for ourselves. A thousand fibres connect us with our fellow men."
> ~ Herman Melville ~

Connection is making a different and deeper joining to all the relationships you have, more compassion, more patience, more understanding, more creativity, and more love.

This makes such a difference in all aspects of your life. You stay true to yourself, your values, your work in the world. You shine your own light so that others can see their own light better.

Love, value, and choices

What are you connected to? This exercise builds on your exploration from all the earlier signposts and gets you thinking about your connection to yourself.

Enjoy, and be curious about what you discover. Don't overthink it.

Find that quiet place and write.

Here's what to do...

Grab a pen, and follow the directions on the next page...

"I love..."

Make a list of everything that comes to you that you love.

Be as specific as possible.

The list may include people, places, things, feelings and activities – anything that comes to mind.

Breathe slowly and sit quietly.

Pay attention to the rise and fall of your body ...

Let your pen write down whatever comes.

I love...

I value..."

Write down all the things you value – the things you feel are important – in your life, your work, and the world.

Be as specific as possible (again).

Write down whatever comes to mind without judgment.

Breathe slowly, and sit quietly, get grounded, go home.

Pay attention to the rise and fall of your body ...

Let your pen write down whatever comes.

I value...

"I spend money on..."   *"I spend time on..."*   &   *"I spend energy on..."*

Now write down what you spend money, time, and energy on…

One after the other, then repeating all three over, and over

Let your hand move on the pages without judgment, you're seeking self-knowledge

I spend...

Money on	Time on	Energy on

Lay all the lists out in front of you, and re-read what you've written

1. How much of your time, energy, and money is spent on the things you love?

2. How much is spent on the things you value?

3. How much is spent on things you neither love nor value?

4. Could you make another choice? Is there anything you could let go of?

5. Do you want, or do you value, things you were not aware of?

6. Are any of these choices based on someone else's values?

7. Are there any choices based on fear?

With compassion, see the choices you're making and the consequences of these choices.

Did you have fun with the process? How did it make you feel? Where are your strongest connections? How much time do you spend on the things that you feel most connected to?

When you're finished, find a place to lie down, relax, take 3 deep breaths in through the nose, and out through the mouth, letting all your thoughts drift away...

If you've been writing in your journal regularly since the first exercise, now is a good time to go back over your journalling from the beginning.

"Journalling is like whispering to one's self and listening at the same time."

~ Mina Murray ~

Notice if, and how, your journalling has changed. Have you changed?

How has paying attention to yourself helped?

Listen closely to what your insights have been whispering.

Follow up on the guidance you've received from yourself.

Is it time to add any actions into your life?

The Wholeness Quest Workbook & Journal

"Writing and reading decrease our sense of isolation.
They deepen and widen and expand our sense of life: they feed the soul."
~ Anne Lamott ~

9. Compassionate

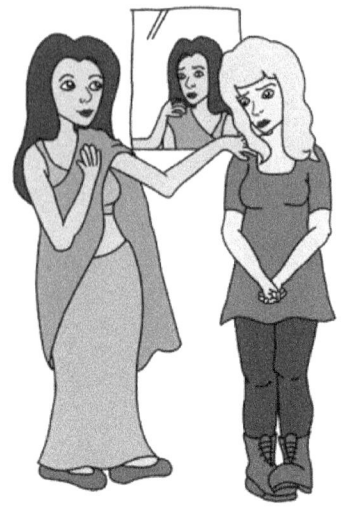

Signpost nine is compassionate.

A strong desire to alleviate the suffering of others.

As you start to get your own life in order, to live the life you choose, you may find that you want to get engaged and go out of your way to help the physical, intellectual, spiritual, or emotional needs of others.

You may want them to benefit from what you've learned, the same way you've benefitted from the learning of others.

Possibly by creating a workbook and journal about your Wholeness Quest…

"Humans are tribal beings, we're motivated by a desire to help, in fact there's good evidence that it's part of our deep evolutionary purpose and vital to the survival of our species".

~ Dasher Keltner ~

People who practice kindness, compassion and self-compassion are happier—the evidence is all there. Here are some of the reasons to practice compassion:

- It makes us feel good
- It activates pleasure circuits and that leads to lasting increases in self-reported happiness
- It reduces the risk of heart disease
- It makes our minds wander less
- It makes us more optimistic and supportive
- It allows us to make better friends with greater satisfaction and growth
- It makes us more positive and less vulnerable to stress and harm to our immune system.

Dacher Keltner tells us about compassion and its particular connection to emotion and action. While some may dismiss it as "touchy-feely or irrational, scientists have started to map the biological basis of compassion, suggesting its deep evolutionary purpose".

Keltner also writes about research showing that when we feel compassion, our heart rate slows down, we secrete the bonding hormone oxytocin, and regions of the brain linked to empathy, caregiving, and feelings of pleasure light up, which often results in our wanting to approach and care for other people.

And here's the segue from connection to compassion.

I love this quote by Charles Darwin...

"A human being is a part of the whole, called by us 'Universe', a part limited in time and space. He experiences himself, his thoughts and feelings as something separated from the rest, a kind of optical delusion of his consciousness.

This delusion is a kind of prison for us, restricting us to our personal desires and to affection for a few persons nearest to us.

Our task must be to free ourselves from this prison by widening our circle of compassion to embrace all living creatures and the whole of nature in its beauty. Nobody is able to achieve this completely, but the striving for such achievement is in itself a part of the liberation and a foundation for inner security."

The good news is that yes, you can practice compassion and get better at it. It's takes the connected signpost to a whole new level.

There are lots of ways to practice, and according to Kristen Neff, the best way to really feel it is to start with self-compassion: self-kindness, common humanity, and mindfulness.

To achieve compassion for yourself, it's time to integrate the old and new you, and don't forget all the beautiful lessons and skills you've discovered throughout this workbook and journal, and on your own Quest.

Practicing kindness and compassion

As I said earlier, the good news is that 'yes' you can practice compassion and get better at it. And remember, when we think we're capable of making a difference, we're less likely to curb our compassion. So, keep building your capability and you'll be able to practice your compassion even more.

Here's what to do...

The key to developing compassion in your life is to make it a daily practice.

3 Compassion Practices

1. ### Morning ritual
   Greet each morning with a ritual. Try this one, suggested by His Holiness, The Dalai Lama:

"Today I'm fortunate to have woken up, I am alive, I have a precious human life, I am not going to waste it. I am going to use all my energies to develop myself, to expand my heart out to others, to achieve enlightenment for the benefit of all beings, I am going to have kind thoughts towards others, I am not going to get angry or think badly about others, I am going to benefit others as much as I can."

What's your ritual greeting for the day going to be?

Then, when you've got your ritual in motion for a day or two, work your way through one of the practices below.

2. *Commonalities practice*

   Instead of recognising the differences between yourself and others, try to recognise what you have in common. At the root of it all, we're all human beings. We need food, and shelter, and love. We crave attention, and recognition, and affection, and above all, happiness. Reflect on these commonalities you have with every other human being, and ignore the differences. One of the best exercises comes from a great article from Ode Magazine — it's a five-step exercise to try when you meet friends and strangers. Do it discreetly and try to do all the steps with the same person. With your attention geared to the other person, tell yourself:

   - Step 1: "Just like me, this person is seeking happiness in her/his/their life."
   - Step 2: "Just like me, this person is trying to avoid suffering in her/his/their life."
   - Step 3: "Just like me, this person has known sadness, loneliness and despair."
   - Step 4: "Just like me, this person is seeking to fill her/his/their needs."
   - Step 5: "Just like me, this person is learning about life."

3. *Evening routine*

   And of course, I highly recommend that you take a few minutes before you go to bed to reflect upon your day. After your recollection of gratitude and how you lived your values, think, and write about the people you met and talked to, and how you treated each other. Think and write about your intention (or the one you use courtesy of the Dalai Lama) that you stated this morning, to act with compassion towards others.

   How well did you do? What could you do better tomorrow? What did you learn from your experiences today?

These compassionate practices can be done anywhere, any time: At work, at home, on the road, while traveling, while at a shop, while at the home of a friend or family member.

By sandwiching your day with a morning and evening ritual, you can frame or bookend your day properly, in an attitude of trying to practice compassion and develop it within yourself.

With practice, you can begin to do it throughout the day, and throughout your lifetime. This will bring happiness to your life and to those around you.

"Compassion is not about weakness.
The ability to show true compassion is neither soft nor touchy feely.
It requires great inner strength, courage, and power.
It is one of greatest gifts one human can bestow on another."
~ Douglas Noll ~

An exercise in self-compassion

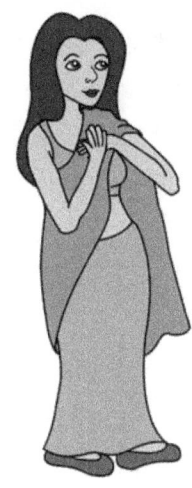

Why not try treating yourself with some compassion, you know you deserve it.

Pay attention—it's your remarkable life.

It's so much easier to be compassionate to another person when you've had the practice with yourself.

Here's what to do...

Take out your journal and answer the following questions:

1. First, think about times when a close friend feels really bad about her or him or themselves or is really struggling in some way. How would you respond to your friend in this situation (especially when you're at your best)?
Write down what you typically do, what you say, and note the tone in which you typically talk to your friends.

2. Now, think about times when you feel bad about yourself or are struggling. How do you typically respond to yourself in these situations? Please write down what you typically do, what you say, and note the tone in which you talk to yourself.

3. Did you notice a difference? If so, ask yourself why. What factors or fears come into play that lead you to treat yourself and others so differently?

4. Now, write down how you think things might change if you responded to yourself in the same way you typically respond to a close friend when you're suffering.

_____
_____
_____
_____
_____

"Tenderness and kindness are not signs of weakness and despair, but manifestations of strength and resolution"
~ Kahlil Gibran ~

"My mission in life is not merely to survive, but to thrive; and to do so with passion, some compassion, some humour and some style"
~ Maya Angelou ~

10. Concordant

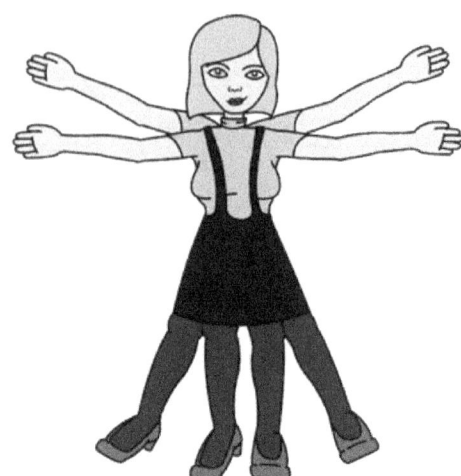

The tenth, and final signpost is concordant.

This beautiful word brings to mind resonance, peaceful, being in agreement, harmonious.

In the end, the thing you want and need is concordance, the state of harmony where all the parts of you are in agreement—body, mind and soul, no more discord. Your life is your own.

From here, growing confidence that you're living your truth takes you to wherever you want to be.

Putting it all together

This is the final exercise in the Wholeness Quest Workbook and Journal, putting it all together.

Create your own declaration for your life, right now.

> "Do you know that our soul is composed of harmony?"
>
> ~ Leonardo da Vinci ~

Here's what to do...

Use the next page or design one of your own. Add colour and pictures if you wish.

Schedule some time to read over your Wholeness Quest Workbook and Journal, and all the exercises you completed.

How far have you come since you began? What changes have you made by paying attention to yourself.

Take three slow deep breaths, perhaps even listen to the Stillness Exercise or your favourite meditation.

Now open your eyes and start to write.

Today I declare...

Even if I'm confused and conflicted, I am grateful for...

I'm conscious that right now I value...

I'm curious, what else is possible? I am becoming...

I'm courageous, I am taking action to...

Keep going...

I'm capable, here's what I can do, and here's what I'm learning next...

I'm closed, and this is how I am taking time out to be...

I'm creative and having fun in these ways...

I'm connected and staying true to myself by...

Almost there...

I'm compassionate and offering the next person a hand up by...

I'm concordant, I practice living in harmony, being me, by...

The final words

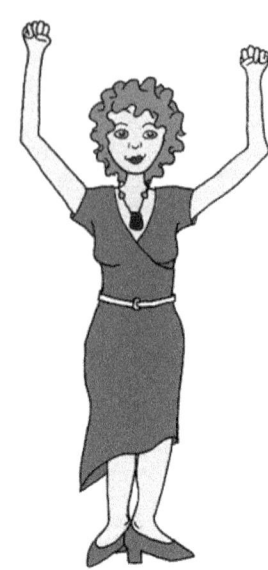

You've done it. Made it to the final words.

I hope you've found that paying attention to yourself has paid off. That you're realising what a remarkable being you are, and what a remarkable life you have.

I love helping people who are searching for fulfillment to find feeling, healing, and reconnection so that they can live a life that expresses the very best they can be.

I had an ordinary and predictable life until the birth and death of my daughter Jacqui Bree. After her death I fell into grief for a long time. Decades later, with the help of two honest friends, I committed to finding a better way to be. Now my life is remarkable, it's worthy of attention... my attention.

I've written myself a new story.

I dream more, I do more, and I'm living the version of myself that expresses the very best of who I can be.

I'm the sum total of all my experiences and choices to this point in time.

Now I work with people who want to make a powerful and compassionate impact on the world. They want to be seen, to be heard, and to make a difference that radically transforms lives.

And I write, four books so far, and lots more to come...

Who do you dream of being? What version of yourself is waiting in the wings?

What does your dream life look, sound, taste, and feel like?

What small step can you take to start living that dream now?

Go on then...

Show Up, Step Up, and offer the person next to you a Hand Up.

Thank you, Veronica xox

Thank you for taking the time to read and reflect in your Wholeness Quest Workbook and Journal. There are some extra pages overleaf for more of your thoughts, insights, and ideas.

If you enjoyed using this book to complete your Quest, please consider taking a moment to write a review on your favourite platform. Even a couple of sentences helps. As an independent author, I rely on reviews and word of mouth.

Your support and feedback are greatly appreciated and can really make a difference. Also, someone else who needs this workbook may find it by reading your review.

If you're ready for a little more help to get yourself on track towards finding your purpose, living and leading consciously and confidently, then you could be ready for My Remarkable Life Online Coaching Program. If you're not sure, there's a free life check-in to try on the website at www.veronicastrachan.com.au/the-program/

If you'd like to discover more about your own strengths, go to Veronica's True Dialogue website (*www.truedialogue.com.au/leadership-coaching/work-with-a-coach/*) and book an Expert Strengths Profile assessment and debrief.

If you haven't already read my memoir Breathing While Drowning: One Woman's Quest for Wholeness, and you'd like to, go here www.veronicastrachan.com.au/breathing-while-drowning/ or you can purchase it from your favourite bookstore.

You'll find the other books that I've written on the website as well, and you can sign up for my irregular newsletter to get updates on my next publication, or follow my blog to read about where I'm up to on my own continuing Quest for Wholeness.

About Veronica Strachan

Veronica Strachan was born to working class parents in the northern suburbs of Melbourne, Australia. The birth of her second daughter who had a severe brain injury changed the direction of Veronica's life forever. The lessons she learnt from Jacqueline Bree's life and death are now her touchstone for living a whole, vibrant, and remarkable life.

From her early career as a nurse and midwife, through evolutions as a project and change manager, CEO and consultant, Veronica now divides her time between writing and coaching remarkable women leaders who want to make a powerful and compassionate impact on the world.

Veronica spent as much of her childhood as she could lost in a good book. She spent most of her adult life lost in a good job as a nurse, midwife, CEO, coach, and facilitator.

"Breathing While Drowning: One Woman's Quest for Wholeness" was her first book. One hundred percent of the sale profits from the book are contributed to Very Special Kids, which operates a hospice for terminally-ill children in Victoria.

Now Veronica and her daughter Cassi have teamed up for a new series *"The Adventures of Chickabella"*. Book 1 is *"Chickabella and the Rainbow Magic"*, which is dedicated to the memory of Veronica's sister, Mary who told the best stories. Book 2 is *"Chickabella Counts to Ten"*. There is at least one more planned in the series, *"Chickabella Shapes Up."*

Under the pen name V. E. Patton, Veronica is currently completing *"Soul Staff: The Opal Dreaming Chronicles Book 2"*, which is due for release in late 2020. *"Ochre Dragon: The Opal Dreaming Chronicles Book 1"* was released in January 2019.

Veronica lives in central Victoria, Australia with her ever-patient husband, one of her three adult children, and a menagerie of animals.

You can find out more about her writing or get in touch via her website www.veronicastrachan.com or follow her on social media: Twitter @truedialogue, Facebook veronicastrachan8, and Instagram @writer_ron.

True Dialogue Publishing

You can find other books and works, including some free stuff at
www.veronicastrachan.com.au

Writing as Veronica Strachan

Memoir

Breathing While Drowning: One Woman's Quest for Wholeness
(paperback ISBN 978-0-6485134-0-7 and ebook ISBN 978-0-6485134-1-4)

Children's Picture Books

Chickabella and the Rainbow Magic
(paperback ISBN 978-0-6485134-3-8 and ebook ISBN 978-0-6485134-2-1)

Chickabella Counts to Ten
(paperback ISBN 978-0-6485134-9-0 and ebook ISBN 978-0-6485134-7-6)

Chickabella Shapes Up (coming soon)

Writing as V. E. Patton

Fantasy

Ochre Dragon : The Opal Dreaming Chronicles Book 1
(paperback ISBN 978-16274739-3-4 and ebook ISBN 978-1-6274734-2-2)

Soul Staff: The Opal Dreaming Chronicles Book 2 (coming 2020)

Short Story Anthology

Peace on Earth in Christmas Australis: A Frighteningly Festive Anthology of Spine Jingling Tales
(paperback ISBN 978-0-6485134-5-2 and ebook ISBN 978-0-6485134-4-5)

www.ingramcontent.com/pod-product-compliance
Lightning Source LLC
Chambersburg PA
CBHW060533010526
44107CB00059B/2628